LIVING FIT AFTER FIFTY

A Guide For the

Post-Menopausal Woman

By

Carol Ann Haines

BEARHEAD PUBLISHING
- BhP -
Brandenburg, Kentucky

BEARHEAD PUBLISHING

- BhP -

Brandenburg, Kentucky
www.bearheadpublishing.com

Living Fit After Fifty
by Carol Ann Haines

Cover Concept by Carol Ann Haines
Cover Arrangement by Aaron S. Haines
Cover Design & Layout by Bearhead Publishing
First Printing - December 2011
ISBN: 978-1-937508-10-4
1 2 3 4 5

Proudly Printed in the United States of America.

LIVING FIT AFTER FIFTY

A Guide For the

Post-Menopausal Woman

Disclaimer

Consult your healthcare professional before beginning any new diet or exercise program. The content of this book is the opinion and personal experience of the author and intended to do no harm. It is not intended to malign any religion, ethnic group, club, organization, company or individual. The author is not responsible for translation, interpretation, bad grammar, or punctuation and is held harmless for any harm.

Foreword

Living Fit after 50 is an upbeat survival guide for people who are at a crossroads--like me. Carol Haines has written a book full of great ideas, solutions and recipes to help navigate this interesting and, at times, irritating stage of life. *Living Fit after 50* provides a positive approach to handling menopause and the assorted goodies that come with middle age, being hijacked by hormones, weight gain, assorted aches and pains, and handling all that life throws your way. Carol's book is written in an easygoing and positive way that make the changes needed in nutrition, exercise and attitude, an easy and doable process. *Living Fit After 50* gives women the confidence to face challenges head on with strength and grace.

 I have had the pleasure of getting to know Carol over the past few years. During this time I have gleaned bits and pieces of her personality and each new discovery is more interesting than the last. I found out she was writing a book in a writing class: kind of cool. She publishes a magazine article: Very cool. She actually finishes her book and has the guts to search out a publisher to share her baby: Outstanding! Who does this kind of thing when you are middle aged and supposedly past your prime? Carol. I've also learned about the many personal struggles that Carol has faced that took courage, determination and sheer will to see through. I admire her daring attitude immensely. This book is optimistic and hopeful, just as Carol is in real life. I can't wait to share this book with my sisters and friends.

Stacey Becker
Star 3 Spinning Instructor
Spinning and Cardio trainer for UCSD Swim Team
Personal Trainer
Mom to 4 sons

Preface

It seems many of my fifty plus female friends and acquaintances are struggling with the symptoms of menopause, specifically the extra pounds we tend to accumulate during and after 'the change.' Despite continuing the diet and exercise programs we followed in the past, this new excess weight is determined to stay with us. Combined with hot flashes, mood swings, and fatigue, we, as a generation of women, are searching for answers. Prior to menopause, I survived a life changing illness, and promised myself I would make the most of the rest of my days. I did not, however, realize my plans would veer off track as menopause approached.

I don't remember my mother, or any of my friends' mothers suffering or complaining about the effects of menopause. Did they just soldier on, quietly accepting the emotional and physical havoc we are unwilling to accept? Today we have more options than they did. We are, or should be, better informed and more proactive regarding our physical and emotional well-being. My search for menopausal relief included: the Internet, bookstores, numerous doctors as well as naturopathic practitioners. I found each source had recommendations relating to their specific area, but I was unable to find a complete program addressing all of the unique needs of post-menopausal women. After years of trial and error, I eventually succeeded in adapting a healthful and energizing program that has allowed me to return to my pre-menopausal weight.

This is the story of my fitness transformation, my decision to live life with vigor and purpose. Some of my post-menopausal friends question me about my weight management plan. They think I don't eat anything, or that I exercise excessively. When I explain I've embarked on a positive lifestyle change, they roll their eyes, imagining a life of starvation and deprivation. Most people think a change like I made would be too complicated, or that it wouldn't work for them. Actually, the opposite is true.

It is my hope that this guide will simplify adapting a healthy lifestyle for my curious friends and anyone else searching for a lifelong fitness plan. This book targets fifty-plus, post-menopausal women, but the plan works for anyone, as my newly fit and trim husband will attest to.

Most of the information in this book relates to physical fitness and dietary changes. The decisions regarding Hormone Replacement Therapy (HRT), Bio Identical Hormone Therapy, or any medical treatments are individual and personal. You, together with your health care professional can explore options and decide if any treatment is appropriate in your case. My philosophy regarding taking medication of any kind comes down to quality of life. If an illness or condition becomes disruptive to my family, work, or general happiness, I consider medication. As a rule I try to stay away from medication, but life is short and if there is help for an unmanageable condition, I will seek it out. You make the choice that is right for you.

What I am sharing here is a lifetime of experiencing what is counter-productive to long-term weight loss and a healthy metabolism, as well as what I have learned from my son who works as a personal fitness trainer, and has taught me how to live well. At the time of this writing I have maintained a healthy weight and body mass index (BMI, amount of body fat) for five years. I eat more than I ever have and do not feel deprived in any way. I enjoy my four times weekly workouts because they keep me strong, flexible, and grounded. I am now ready for any and all adventures.

This well-rounded fitness program consists of four parts: mental attitude, diet, strength training to maintain healthy muscles and cardiovascular exercise for fat loss. I learned that all of the elements of the plan are necessary for fifty something post-menopausal women who, like me are struggling like never before to remain or become fit. Mental attitude is by far the most important part, because without the right attitude, you are setting yourself up for failure. Most of us have experienced enough diet failures to last a lifetime, so let's change gears and enjoy success!

Chapter 1

Motivation

Deciding to Live

The look on my surgeon's face told me more than any words could convey. Despite his best efforts to remain composed there was no denying he was anxious about my biopsy results. It was confirmed. The lump under my arm was melanoma, a cancer for which there is no cure. Nine years after a cancerous mole was removed from my forearm the disease had once again raised its ugly head.

For the last 17 years I had lived with a subconscious fear of melanoma. The big 'C' first invaded my life during my first pregnancy, at the age of thirty, when I had a thin mole removed from my face. It was diagnosed as malignant melanoma, but in its early stage. I was told it should not cause any more problems; however, I was instructed to remain vigilant of any changes to my skin. Then at 38, another primary melanoma was removed from my right forearm. This time it was slightly deeper, but probably caught in time. With my naturally optimistic attitude, I assumed that probably meant I was done with skin cancer, and filed my fears away in the far reaches of my mind.

Now, with the diagnosis that the cancer was back, and had entered my blood stream, my husband Mark and I returned home with surgery schedules, an oncologist's phone number and despair in our hearts. I was 47 and our two sons were in their teens. Would I be here to see them grow up? I believed in my heart that I would. I just had to be. Within a month the tumor was removed and I was faced with an agonizing decision. The survival rate for stage III melanoma is not very good and I was instructed to undergo adjuvant treatment (chemotherapy). However, the one FDA approved course of treatment for melanoma was a year long, with multiple side effects and not much improvement in the survival numbers. My instincts guided me to search for a better plan to fight this battle. For the next few weeks, while I healed from the surgery, I spent sleepless nights on the Internet researching drug trials. Desperation drove me on, and eventually I found a trial that I was able to put all my faith in, and treatment was scheduled.

The treatment consisted of a cocktail of toxic drugs, three hospital stays, extreme nausea, high fevers, and depression. These months were literally the worst of my life. I had never been so sick and the reality of dying was very prominent in my mind. Through the lonely hours lying in bed sick and drugged, I never lost the will to live. I wanted my health back, to be able to do the routine everyday chores I was unable to do. I even wished I could get up and do the laundry, something I had always hated.

By the third month I was unable to hold anything down and spent more time at the hospital. I did not know if I was strong enough to complete the course of treatment. My doctor expressed the importance of my finishing the treatment to my husband, and he supported and encouraged me to continue for the sake of our family.

Yes, I would continue, and I would survive. I made up my mind that I was going to get through this challenge, regain my strength, and live out my life to the fullest. I promised myself I would appreciate every day (even laundry day). I would accept all invitations, I would welcome adventure, I would travel, and I would love and cherish my family and friends.

Finally it was over. No more poisoning drugs, no more throwing up, but a long road to recovery. As my system began to accept food, I gradually got stronger and greeted every day with joy. I was ecstatic to be able to do more of the things I had missed. I was caring for my family, going out, and I was gaining weight.

Before I was diagnosed with cancer, I had been 10 to 15 pounds overweight, not so unusual for a 47-year-old woman. Now, a year after completing the treatment, I was 30 pounds overweight. I was fat. The months of eating next to nothing had triggered my body into survival mode and unbeknownst to me it was packing away fat for future illness or self-imposed famines (fad diets). The images I had of myself living life to the fullest during my illness were of a healthy, strong woman. Now I was being dragged down by this excess weight and not finding the adventure and happiness I had promised myself. It was time to take action.

I inherited the tendency to carry extra weight and over the years had tried every fad diet that came along. Actually, I had been on one diet or another since I was 18. Over the next several years I revisited all those restrictive diets: low carbohydrate, no carbohydrate, low fat, no fat, low calorie and eventually, hardly any calories at all. I exercised as I had in the past but was not getting the same results. I might lose a little each time I switched diets, but I would gain the lost weight back and became convinced that I was destined to be overweight. At age 54 the image I had of conquering the world was fading. I was staying home more; hated shopping for clothes, and was not appreciating or enjoying life as I had promised myself.

In the meantime, my oldest son, Ryan, had begun a career as a personal trainer. He was aware of my struggle and suggested I stop starving myself and commit to a six-week program with him. Well, I couldn't imagine that my kid could know more about my metabolism than I did and I balked at the idea. He would require that I work out five times a week, which was fine, eat six times a day, and stay off the scale for the entire six weeks. Eat all that food and not weigh myself? I thought he was crazy and told him I knew I couldn't eat like that. He then asked me how my program was working for me, and I had to admit, it wasn't. "Mom," he said. "You conquered cancer, you can conquer a few pounds of fat."

Chapter 2

Attitude

What's Your Excuse?

I have used them all: it's hereditary, I'm too busy, I have bad knees, I can't afford a trainer. Each of these excuses for not following a healthy lifestyle has some merit. Let's address them as they relate to me. Everyone in my immediate family is fat. One of my brothers was a skinny child, but now at midlife, even he has the non-beer drinker's beer belly. It is an extra challenge when you carry the fat gene, but lots of people do. The tendency to be fat can be conquered. The question is, are you willing to make the changes necessary to overcome it? You may already eat very little and blame your metabolism for being overweight. Consider that a slow metabolism could be your body's reaction to not eating enough.

Everyone is busy. Finding time to exercise might seem impossible, but where there's a will, there's a way. Get up earlier, or extend your lunch break on workout days. Move dinner back an hour a few times a week. Many busy people make time to exercise, and you can too. If you raised kids, worked full time, managed a home, sometimes on your own, you can certainly find time to exercise. By this age our kids are older and less reliant on us, freeing up some 'me' time. Make the most of this time. You've earned it.

After fifty, most of us have aches and pains from old injuries, surgeries, and/or arthritis. I suffered a severe whiplash when I was 26 and it continues to plague me. Additionally, both of my knees were injured in that same accident. One was surgically repaired and the other became my 'weak' knee until I blew out its ACL in a skiing mishap. After I had the ACL reconstructed, this knee became my 'good' knee. Luckily for me this skiing accident occurred at a major resort with experienced Sports Medicine Orthopedic doctors on hand. They got me up immediately (and I mean immediately) to begin exercising the repaired knee. At the time I thought it was insanity to be in the therapy room hours after surgery. Now I am very grateful to my surgeon, who pushed me to exercise that knee when I thought I should be in bed recuperating. This experience taught me that strong muscles and flexibility protect and support weak or previously injured joints. Exercise lessens the effects of aging and should not be shied away from. As my mom used to say "Use it or lose it". The more time you spend sitting, the faster you will age.

We all know you can't buy happiness. The same is true for fitness. A trainer is a wonderful coach, but unless you commit to a well-rounded program and do the work, you will fail again and again. Invest in yourself. You can make it happen. With or without a trainer, it's about you taking control of your own well being. If you have the means to hire a trainer, find a good one. Like anything else, there are bad apples in the trainer barrel. Ask around, check credentials and experience, and ask to speak to some of your prospective trainer's clients. Even a few sessions with a trainer is a great way to learn how to use the equipment properly. Correct form is extremely important for getting results and avoiding injury. This knowledge will increase the effectiveness of your workouts tremendously. If you are not able to work with a trainer, you can learn and succeed on your own. Exercise options are everywhere. The stairs in your house, the community pool, exercise DVDs, are all great places to start. That dusty bicycle in the garage or the walking shoes in your closet will get you outdoors and in the sunshine. My point here is that all your excuses are just that, excuses. Unless you have a major physical impairment, you really don't have a valid reason to neglect your physical health.

Life is full of choices and hopefully we make the right ones most often. You can choose to continue a less healthy life-style by being overweight, out of shape and heading for an early rocking chair, which is fine if you are content and happy. Or you can say no to that rocking chair and yes to increased energy, better health, and probably a longer life. No more excuses.

Think Positively

You can kick your metabolism into high gear and train it to burn calories for energy instead of packing them away in the form of fat. I did not believe it was true for us post-menopausal women, but the proof is in the results. Our bodies are very smart and built for survival. Years of fad dieting have trained our bodies to store fat. You can teach your body to change for the better. I have done it, and it is easier than I ever thought possible. Give your body what it needs! It needs fuel to function normally and to maintain its healthy tissue. Is there anything that runs well without fuel? I don't think so. Starving gives us the undesirable result of slowing our metabolism down which is our survival instinct at work.

The first step towards achieving this change is to forget all our old ideas about dieting. Let it go! Accept that you may be wrong. If you are able to maintain your perfect weight and body mass index, then you do know all you need to know about dieting. If you yo-yo diet or struggle to be in the kind of shape you dream of, then maybe you don't. I was sure that carbohydrates made me fat. Ryan kept telling me that I was not eating enough. I told him I was sensitive to carbohydrates and couldn't eat them. He pointed out to me that carbohydrates are our bodies' energy source.

"How do you expect your body to function efficiently without the proper fuel?" he asked. "Why not open your mind to a positive change?" I had all the answers, but no results to prove my theories. Change of any kind can be difficult for our age group, as well as admitting that we are wrong. In fact, making dietary and exercise changes is the hardest part of adapting a healthy lifestyle. Someone diagnosed with a life threatening condition can usually make the changes necessary to save their life. This shows us that with the right motivation or attitude, we can change our habits and behaviors. Once the new routine is established it is not hard at all. And, getting results is a great motivator.

Thinking of your new nutrition-plan as a diet may sabotage your good intentions. We all hate the restrictions and failure associated with our past dieting efforts. Diets don't work. Over the short term they may work quite well, but you are not likely to stay on a restrictive diet forever. Soon, after resuming your normal diet, you will begin to regain that lost weight along with some bonus fat for your body to store for your next restrictive diet. The yo-yo diet weight losses and regains are not healthy, physically or mentally. Too many weight fluctuations can put stress on your heart, and failure is depressing.

Start thinking in terms of what you need to eat for good health instead of what you can't eat. Focusing on the positive aspect of any challenge will make it easier. I am always thinking ahead to my next meal or snack, which is never more than three hours away. This does not leave a lot of time to worry about those cookies I 'can't' have. Your body needs to be fed regularly and frequently, so think about what it will need next and your bad eating habits may resolve themselves.

Put the vision of a strong, lean woman in your mind, and your chances of becoming one are more likely to be realized. Replace the negative self-images we tend to carry with us with positive ones. Visualization is a powerful weapon to keep in your arsenal. When you are feeling discouraged, picture a healthy new you, standing tall, being fit, and living with vitality. The image will inspire you to take care of yourself and your mind will begin to change its concept of who you are.

You will have meltdowns from time to time, which is not the end of the world. Be accepting of yourself. Don't undermine your progress with guilt and disappointment. Having dessert occasionally is not a crime. Realize that you are human and when you falter, get back on that horse and ride on. Once you have retrained your body to use calories for energy, you should be able to metabolize dessert now and then. Everything in moderation, including moderation, is a good motto to live by. This plan is about a happier, healthier, more active life. Focus on the benefits and be proud of yourself for each positive change. Treat your body right and it will return the favor.

Managing Stress

When life is dumping on you from all sides, do you find yourself reaching for carbohydrate-laden munchies? If you do, you are reacting to another human instinct to protect yourself. We are programmed to increase fat storage at times of stress in order to survive famine or do battle. I doubt that any of us will ever face either of these circumstances, but we all have different, very real, modern day stresses. However, we will not be going into battle to use up that stored survival fat. The consequences are weighty (literally) if we continually subject ourselves to unmanaged stress.

Carrying anxiety with you from one crisis to the next puts stress on you physically as well as mentally. And does the worry and anxiety solve any problem or crisis? No. Instead it clouds your mind and skews your rational thought process, which you need command of during times of trouble. Let's turn all of that energy towards finding paths to acceptance.

So how do we handle all of life's challenges? First we must all accept that life is uncertain and will never be problem free. All that we experience and endure makes us who we are. Learning to face life's trials, both large and small, with grace and composure is important for your overall wellness. In other words, don't sweat the small stuff, and it's all small stuff.

You may have a hard time considering your crisis of the week as small stuff, but in the grand scheme of things, it probably is. Do you still have a roof over your head? Is your family relatively healthy and safe? Do you have something to eat and water to drink? If your answer to these questions is yes, then you are going to be fine. You will get through whatever is happening and be stronger and wiser for it. The world isn't ganging up on you, its just life. Unfortunately we will all face some very real, devastating tragedies that only time will heal, but with the right frame of mind you will find the strength and composure to get you through.

Developing the habit of meditating on a regular basis can ground you and give you a fresh perspective when dealing with your daily dilemmas. It does not have to be time consuming or burdensome. Make it simple and enjoyable. When stress takes control of you and you can't be alone, try taking some deep breaths. Think about your breathing for a few seconds and imagine the oxygen strengthening your being. This simple technique may save you from losing your cool, and maybe your job. When you are at home, or on a break, find a quiet space, preferably outside, and let nature nourish your spirit. Focus all your attention on a bee, busy with a flower, or a spider spinning a web. Even the movement of leaves in the breeze can take you away to that meditative state. If you are inside, close your eyes and focus on sound, music or rain falling, and remember to breathe. Experiment and discover what brings you a few minutes of peace.

My favorite way to alleviate stress is laughter. Watching a comedy, or calling a jokester friend that always makes me laugh is effective, inexpensive therapy. Another method that has helped me tremendously is to UNPLUG once in a while. By this I mean turning off the TV, putting down the cell phone, shutting down the computer, even your ipod. This constant stream of information, coming from a multitude of sources, is stressing our brains without our realizing it. A few hours each week without any electronic signals coming at you is like a vacation. At first you may feel a little lost, but soon you are noticing birds and flowers and the weather. It really is quite nice. I highly recommend it.

You will be doing your waistline and your sanity a favor if you adopt the glass-half-full attitude and roll with the punches of everyday life. Worrying and stressing will not solve anything.

Set a Goal and Take Control

You do have the power to change your body. Have you ever read the Serenity Prayer? It's the prayer that asks God to help you change the things you can, accept the things you can't, and the wisdom to know the difference. Health and fitness are largely in our control to change. Much of our ill health is related to our lifestyle and the choices we make regarding diet and exercise. It goes without saying that smoking and excessive alcohol consumption is detrimental to our health. Most people accept this, but too many of us do not consider a poor diet and a sedentary lifestyle to be as influential to our overall health as they actually are. This is really common sense. Your mother was so very right when she told you to eat your vegetables and go out and play. Instead we rely on fast food and processed meals that contain very little real nutrition. The results of this neglect accumulate over the years and by middle age we are fat, sick and tired. It does not have to be this way.

It's up to you. Make the decision to live well. Picture yourself fit and energetic, ready for all life has to offer. You are too young to stop living. Facing my mortality was a turning point in my life. I learned to value my time and am now determined to get the most out of living and go for the gusto. Shouldn't everyone think like that? We have no way of knowing when life will suddenly change or end. Good health and fitness is your key to getting the most out of each and every day.

If you think you are ready to make this major commitment to yourself, do some mental preparation. Maybe you have a class reunion coming up or a milestone birthday or anniversary. Put that date out there and picture yourself celebrating the occasion looking and feeling really good. Or think about wearing a stylish bathing suit on your next summer vacation. You may balk at the bathing suit idea, but you can make it happen! Be realistic regarding results at our age. We are not super models or movie stars. We are real, middle aged, beautiful women. Nothing looks better on us than good muscle tone, glowing skin and a bright smile. Whatever your particular fitness goal is, you have the power to make it happen! Begin your program with the attitude that you are going to succeed and you will. There is no place in this program for doubts and negative energy. All your energy will be going towards your goal of liking yourself and feeling strong and vital. You are in control.

Chapter 3

Diet

Food – Nourishment for Body and Soul

Our ancestors never dreamed there would come a time when too much food was our nation's biggest health problem. The majority of Americans are overweight. Even 'poor' people are overweight. I am personally grateful to be living in a country where food is plentiful. But overindulgence can undermine our health as surely as malnutrition.

As members of the baby boom generation, we are the first to experience this new relationship with food. Generations before us spent most of their time and efforts securing food for survival. The twentieth century brought mass production and transportation, making food accessible to almost everyone in the United States. Our hardworking ancestors ate a lot, and even though we are much less active today, food remains the central focus of our lives. Celebrations and family gatherings always revolve around food: holiday dinners, backyard barbeques, pot lucks and so on. And what is wrong with that? What is wrong is that most of us do not work physically anymore and do not require the amount of calories even our parents required. We sit at our desks, we order pizza and watch TV. Our lifestyles have changed, but has our diet changed to properly meet our lower caloric requirements?

For some of us food is now the enemy. It's everywhere waiting to catch us off guard. We feel guilty when we eat, but then eat more to console ourselves. Some of us accept weight gain as a normal part of aging. A lot of us struggle to choose between a healthy weight and all the great food and drink available to us everywhere we go, never finding that perfect balance.

Some of my fifty-something friends eat next to nothing. I used to be among this group. They manage to keep their weight relatively low, but they all have an unhealthy body mass index. Some of them are what my trainer son, Ryan, refers to as 'skinny fat'. Even though they appear thin or average size, their body mass index consists of much more fat than it should. This is the result of starving their bodies of the fuel and nutrients it needs to function optimally, burning muscle for energy and storing fat for survival.

'Eat less and exercise more', has been drilled into our heads for years. Our age group grew up being compared to actresses and unnaturally skinny models starting with Twiggy, the first supermodel, who burst on the scene in 1966. Our initial reaction was shock at her thinness, but soon every magazine cover was graced with another skeletal figure wearing the latest fashion. Gaunt and undernourished was the new beautiful. We read in fashion magazines that these glamorous young girls maintained their svelte physiques by surviving on coffee and cigarettes. We all wanted to look like them, and they became our role models. We put ourselves through all kinds of restrictive and unhealthy diets to obtain and maintain our weight. Weight was the only thing that mattered. We gave no thought to health, body composition or even if we looked good. As long as we were thin, we were happy.

Now that we are over fifty we are not getting the results we used to on the starvation plan. Our muscles are shrinking and we are getting saggy and baggie. We're not as thin as we want to be either. It's time to grow up and realize that looking and feeling good comes from being fit and healthy. Being thin (skinny fat) is not the best look for a fifty plus year old woman. Muscle loss makes us look old and frail. There is nothing more youthful looking than a defined and sculpted body. Your body needs materials to build and maintain muscle tissue, so we have to eat! Eating is not a bad thing. It's wonderful to be able to eat and not gain weight. But you must retrain your body to utilize the food that you eat instead of storing it as fat.

One day, in reference to one of his clients, Ryan asked me, "How do I get a 45-year old woman to eat? She refuses to follow the diet plan I recommend for her, and she is not getting results. Why would someone spend the money for a trainer and not follow the plan?"

"Remember how I resisted eating everything you recommended at first?" I asked. "Tell her about me. Show her my before and after pictures." Hearing about my success inspired her to finally follow her nutrition plan and now she is doing great.

Food is good for us and we need it! We need to start thinking more about food and not running away from it. Our focus should be on what we need to eat, not what we can't eat. Planning menus, shopping and preparing food can be therapeutic. Going through the motions of caring for your physical needs is mentally nourishing. As Martha Stewart would say, "It's living". Try thinking of meal preparation as creative and artistic, as opposed to a chore, and as a way of bringing family and friends together for a break from our busy lives. Changing your relationship with food to a positive one will help insure long-term lifestyle changes.

The benefits of healthy eating are far reaching. In addition to less body fat, you will also improve your digestion. Fruits and vegetables (including lots of greens), whole grains and nuts will keep your digestive system functioning smoothly and regularly. You may also experience better sleep, and a good night's sleep is essential if you want to lose weight. Eating whole foods often helps to keep your blood sugar balanced. Say goodbye to sugar highs and lows. Balanced blood sugar also improves your mental attitude. Eventually you may see your blood pressure and cholesterol numbers lower, allowing you to get off medications. Look for your taste buds to change also. They will wake up to the nuances and complexities of natural foods. After several months of eating more raw foods, I noticed I was enjoying them so much more. I never considered fruit a dessert, but now I find it sweet and satisfying. Refined sweets and baked goods have lost their appeal to me. Sugar and white flour tastes bland and boring, absolutely not worth the calories, (chocolate being the exception). Last but not least, shopping! Buying clothes that actually fit well and look good is really fun.

Today I look at food with a fresh new attitude. I look forward to preparing a healthy meal that will fill me up and nourish my body. In the summer I plant a small garden and find being among the fresh plants and sweet herbs replenishes my spirit and energy after a tiring workday. Knowing that I am about to prepare a meal that will be beneficial to body and mind brings joy to the experience. Fresh and natural has become more desirable to me than sugary and processed. What a wholesome change.

Prepare Yourself and Your Pantry

If you are a sugar addict like I was, you will need to find a way to kick the sugar habit. I found myself craving sweets every afternoon and kept a supply of cookies and candies in my pantry for these attacks. Somehow I sort of ignored these calories and did not acknowledge them as the culprit behind my weight gain. Before I committed to a fitness program, I knew I would have to deal with this issue. I devised a plan to replace the sweet snacks with other 'forbidden' foods for a week or so. I allowed myself to choose something else I loved, but was considered off limits to dieters, as long as it wasn't a sweet. I indulged in nuts of all kinds (cashews being my favorite), cheese and crackers, peanut butter, chips and dip, or whatever struck my fancy. I thoroughly enjoyed these high calorie treats for about 10 days, during which time I gradually lost the craving for sugar! Once free of this very real addiction, I felt empowered and ready to take control of the rest of my diet. Whatever your weakness is, mastering it before you begin your program will give you confidence to move forward without any doubts about your commitment.

Clean out your pantry, and any stashes you might have in drawers or cabinets at work. Get rid of all the junk food that will tempt you in a weak moment. If it's not there, you can't eat it. Replenish your shelves with healthy, low calorie foods and snacks. I have included low calorie snack suggestions and recipes that I enjoy at the end of this book. Collect your own recipes from friends who eat light, from magazines, the Internet, books, or discover your own sources.

Invest in a good food scale. A digital scale with grams and ounces is a great tool. You will be surprised how much you use it and will soon learn what your desired portions look like. Find calorie guides online or at your local bookstore. You are then armed with the knowledge you need to navigate menus and buffets. Being prepared in this way will help you get through your transition to a healthy lifestyle.

Consider forming some new habits. Visit your local farmers market each week for good organic produce. Better yet, plant a garden if you have the space. As I mentioned earlier, gardening is a peaceful and rewarding hobby. I have learned to season food with fresh herbs and spices. You can make delicious sauces using juices instead of fat. It just takes a little research and experimenting. Eating light can be delicious.

We all have different schedules and lifestyles, so make a plan that works with yours. Make your program workable for you, a plan that you can stay with for the long haul. Your transition will take a little time, but it will get easier with each passing week. And you will be feeling and looking better, and that is worth making some changes.

What to Eat and When to Eat It

How many times have we heard that breakfast is the most important meal of the day? And how many of us busy working women actually eat breakfast? Now we are being told that eating frequent small meals will increase our metabolism. Guess what? It works. And because your meals are smaller, your stomach will shrink and make over-eating uncomfortable. Starting your day with a nutritious breakfast, breaking your nightly fast, will give your body the signal to start functioning. The sooner you give your body its fuel, the better. Why not start your engines first thing rather than telling your body to continue to conserve energy while it waits for fuel?

But what should I eat, and how much? This is where many 'dieters' turn to the latest fad diet or an old one they have followed before. If those old diet experiences and fad diets worked, you wouldn't be searching for a new one. Each time you lose weight through a strict diet you are slowing down your metabolism. And when you begin to eat more calories, your body will convert them into fat more efficiently than ever. A restrictive diet will eventually lead you right back here, looking for a better diet to lose the weight you regained. Enough already. It's time to do it right.

Let's start with a few basics. To really know how much you are eating, you have to count calories. To determine how many calories your body needs, multiply your current weight by ten, then round the total off to the nearest hundred[1]. I

---

1. Cynthia Sass, R.D. nutritionist and Shape Magazine contributing editor. The Firm, Body Sculpting System 2

weighed approximately 150 pounds when I started so my weight loss plan allowed for 1500 calories per day. For healthy, steady fat loss, it is important to get these calories regularly. If you eat less than your goal weight multiplied by ten, you are telling your metabolism to slow down. This is not the message we want to send. Instead, tell your body it will be receiving what it needs on a regular basis so it will be free to burn the fat while preserving your precious muscle tissue. My goal weight was 125 pounds, which would require 1,250 calories. As you lose weight, you can adjust your total calories, but never go below your goal weight calorie number. So I started with 1500 calories a day and after I lost ten pounds I went to 1400 a day. I did not go lower because I was still losing steadily.

I had no idea what 1500 calories looked like. I learned it could consist of an abundance of healthy food or a very small amount of high calorie junk food. Once you have decided to get healthy and lean, make the commitment to yourself to make the right choices. If you choose high calorie, high fat foods, you won't get much volume. If you choose whole grains, lean protein, fruits, and especially vegetables, you will be surprised at the amount of food you can eat. You don't have to feel hungry or deprived if you eat well. Count all calories. An uncounted bite here and there will add up and sabotage your results. Going cold turkey is the best way to start. Stick to the plan you establish for yourself.

I would be remiss not to mention the importance of water. Thirst can mimic hunger, so satisfy this need with lots of plain water. You can flavor it with lemon or lime, but I recommend cutting out the diet sodas and artificially sweetened drink mixes. The artificial sweeteners may increase your appetite and craving for those sugar calories your body thinks it should be getting from the artificially sweetened drinks. Plus the controversy over the long-term effects of these artificial sweeteners is enough to make me leery of them. I am no dietitian, but where there is smoke there may be fire. My research has led me to choose Stevia, a plant based sweetener, when I want one. This is a personal choice, as artificial sweeteners have little to no calories, but I strive to make the healthiest choices I can.

Eating six times a day may sound time consuming, but with the proper planning and preparation your frequent meals will become routine. Once your metabolism begins to burn more calories your body will let you know when it is time to eat. I began with 1500 calories a day so I will use this number when giving examples of meals and snacks. When you make your personal plan, adjust up or down to meet your daily caloric requirement.

My weight loss program consists of a 300-calorie breakfast and lunch, 450-calorie dinner, and three 150-calorie snacks, approximately 1500 calories. To maintain my goal weight I can increase my calories to 2000 without regaining. Too many days going over 2000 will put the weight back on, so I try to stay a little below 2000. On workout days I eat a little more. On sedentary days it is easy to eat light because I am not as hungry. I eat approximately every three hours. If I am busy and not noticing the time, my stomach will alert me to fuel up right on schedule. In the past I could go for many hours without ever getting hungry. What a difference a functioning metabolism makes. I get ravishingly hungry now if I go past a scheduled meal or snack. My body has actually burned my last meal efficiently and is signaling for fuel. Great, I get to eat again!

Protein, Carbohydrates and Fat

Include Them All

Carbohydrates have been given a bad rap. When eaten in their natural state they provide the energy you need to live an active life. Whole grains, brown and wild rice, and even potatoes should be part of a healthy diet. It is when these foods are processed and refined, or loaded up with butter or gravy, that they become our enemy. In their whole form, carbohydrates burn slowly, giving your body time to use them for energy. If they are refined, the body quickly processes them before it has had time to utilize their calories, and they get converted to, and stored as fat.

Whenever possible choose fresh, raw, organic fruits, vegetables, and grains. Many fruits and vegetables are portable and ready to go. It is just as easy to grab an apple, as it is a cookie or prepackaged snack that may be full of refined sugar, fat and chemicals. Carbohydrates also assist the body in efficiently metabolizing protein. Eating protein and carbohydrates together gives your body all the nutrients it needs to stay strong and active. Unlike fat, the body does not store protein, so it should be consumed in small portions every 2-3 hours to build and maintain healthy tissue. By following the six-meals-a-day plan, you will automatically meet these needs. Choose lean meats, poultry and fish, fat free milk, yogurt and cottage cheese. Beans, nuts, seeds and protein powders and bars, provide variety and portability. Yes, you can and should eat nuts. Just be mindful of the portion and munch away.

Nuts and seeds are a great way to get your daily requirement of healthful essential unsaturated fatty acids. Fats provide steady-burning fuel that staves off hunger to get you through the afternoon without going into a slump. They are also delicious and satisfying. Using limited amounts of olive oil for dressings and marinades will round out your fat requirement. Fats should comprise about 20% of your diet and I find I can stay within this guideline easily enough if I choose unrefined foods and watch my portions.

The most important thing to take from this chapter is the reality of our body's survival instinct. Our bodies will make the necessary adjustments to our metabolism if they fear famine and/or starvation. When we severely restrict calories and nutrients we begin to burn away our healthy muscle tissue and hoard fat for an emergency energy supply, which we will never need. This is the opposite of what we want to tell our bodies. Let your body know that food is plentiful by feeding it regularly. Soon it will realize it can burn that stored fat without fear and your transformation will begin.

Before you head out on your weekly marketing, plan your menus and snacks and make a list. Stock the panty and refrigerator with lots of nutritious food and feel good about eating. Continually remind yourself that you are choosing to live strong and long. If you are in your fifties, you may have thirty or forty years ahead of you. Personally I am choosing to get all I can out of these years. I want to travel, ski, and hike, and I want to feel good while I'm doing all the activities I choose to do. We are too young to stop living. Feed your body right and go for the gusto!

Chapter 4

Weight Training

Why Do It?

You may believe, like I did, that weight training will make you bigger, adding unwanted bulk. Realistically, women, especially post-menopausal women, do not have the hormones required to build large muscles. We have to work hard to build, or even maintain muscle. So why, you may ask, do we want muscles anyway? The obvious answer is that they look good on us. A toned and sculpted body looks strong and youthful. After age thirty-five, the average woman who does not exercise loses one half pound of muscle each year. In addition she will gain a pound of fat each year unless she modifies her diet and exercise patterns[1]. The result is a soft, saggy, fragile body more suited to the rocking chair then the ski slopes or any type of active lifestyle. What did we do to deserve this fate? It doesn't seem fair. The good news is we have the power to change it.

In addition to looking good on us, muscles burn calories. Experts agree muscles burn more calories than fat. More importantly muscle is more metabolically active than fat. Muscle requires energy to move and work. Therefore, challenging

---

1.   The Firm

your muscle mass with weight bearing contractions on a regular basis can result in fat loss[1].

When you lift weights, you are essentially tearing down your muscles. Your body responds immediately after your workout, expending energy to repair and build even stronger muscles. This is part of the, EPOC, or excess post-exercise oxygen consumption, also known as the after-burn. There are many processes occurring after a strenuous weight-training workout to return the body to pre-workout condition. The body must restore glycogen to depleted muscles. It must restore blood lactate levels and bring down its heart rate and body temperature. These processes require energy (calories) and can take hours to complete, extending the benefits of your workout throughout your day. The more intense the workout, the more calories burned during EPOC[2].

Then there are those feel good hormones released during exercise that cause some people to become addicted to the gym. Becoming a gym rat is not our objective here, but the endorphins, serotonin and dopamine released during exercise, are mood boosters. If you are feeling down or have a slight case of the blues, a tough workout is good, natural medicine. And once you begin to see improvement in your strength and physique, a snowball of positive energy keeps you coming back. Starting your day with a trip to the gym, a walk or run outside, or any type of exercise, can put you in a fresh frame of mind. The elevated endorphins flowing through your brain may make you more energetic, more productive, and happier. Some days I feel empowered and proud after completing a strenuous workout. At 58 I am stronger then I have ever been, which makes life more enjoyable. Stairs are now my friends, and lifting and carrying grocery bags is nothing. Bending and

---

1.   Dr. Cedric Bryant, American Council on Exercise
2.   Dr. Cedric Bryant, American Council on Exercise

stooping in my garden brings me joy as opposed to moans and groans and an aching back.

Speaking of an aching back, a strong properly nourished body will lessen the effects of arthritis and over used joints. I have suffered many injuries over the years and have been told by doctors that I would have arthritis in these sites and should be easy on them. However a sports orthopedist may give a different prognosis. When I ended up with my head buried in snow, and my legs tangled in skies that did not release, I knew I was in big trouble. While the ski patrol lifted me onto the basket for transport off the mountain, they reassured me this was the best place to be if you are going to blow out your knees. "We have the best orthopedic surgeons in the world here at Vail. They repair knees and shoulders all day long. We have both had our knees repaired here and we are as good as new." Well, I guessed that was reassuring.

As I waited for my surgery, everyone from the pharmacist to the janitor at the hospital told me they had had their knee, or knees, repaired there, and I would be back on the slopes in no time. I had my doubts as I lay there with one knee screaming in pain and the other one as big as a basketball.

I was wheeled in for my ACL reconstruction about 8:00 pm and was perplexed to be awakened in my room at 7:00 am the very next morning by the physical therapist informing me it was time to get up and head down for my first session of the day. I explained he must be mistaken as I had just had my surgery late last night. He was quite sure I was his patient and proceeded to assist me out of bed and through an obstacle course consisting of stairs and ramps on our way to therapy. I was not a happy camper at this point, but sure enough, I was skiing again ten months later.

I was sent home to San Diego with instructions to follow up with a sports medicine orthopedist and continue therapy to strengthen my legs. It has been close to twenty years since this incident and I continue to work my legs hard, keeping the muscles surrounding and supporting my knees strong.

When I have stopped exercising for periods of time I find that my knees become weak and painful. They do not like the extra load they must carry when my leg muscles are less supportive.

This, and a series of other incidents have taught me that strong muscles are important to protect joints and old injuries. For those of us who choose to remain active during this stage of life, strong muscles are key. I am not recommending that you start working out immediately after an injury or surgery. All injuries are different and you should always follow your physicians' instructions. But once you are given the OK, gradually begin to regain lost strength and eventually build strong and supportive muscles. Your future body will thank you for it.

Form and Technique

It is very common to see people at the gym using the equipment improperly. Don't try to learn proper form and technique by watching others work out. In addition to exercising inefficiently, they are at risk of injuring themselves. Posture and stance is key to getting the most out of your weight lifting workout and protecting your joints and muscles from injury. If you are at a gym, have one of the trainers show you how to use the equipment properly. Don't be shy about asking for help. If you purchased a gym membership I am sure the sales person told you the trainers would be at your disposal. Once they get your money though, you may rarely see a trainer on the floor. Make an appointment if necessary to get the help you need. The best case would be to hire a trainer for at least a few sessions to learn the basics. I would do a little investigating before choosing a trainer, as you want to get the most for your money. Look at the trainers' credentials, how long they have been training, and if possible talk to current clients. Ask people at the gym you see working with trainers if they would recommend their trainer. An informed decision can make a world of difference.

If you are exercising at home or on your own, I recommend DVDs. There are hundreds of great workouts and some really good instructors to choose from. They are not too expensive and can be fun. You will also need to purchase some dumbbells to start with and as you get stronger you may want to include a barbell, step, ankle weights, or any number of tools recommended for the workouts you choose. If you are like me, over time you may amass a small library of DVDs. I have all types and all the equipment to go with them. It's great to have this option for when I don't have time or just don't feel like going to the gym. And mixing up your workouts increases results.

Start with some beginner level workouts if you are not used to exercising, and if you choose to start at home with a DVD, view the entire workout first. Watch the instructor/ instructors and learn the moves, proper stance, and posture. I like to imagine a chain is attached to my head and pulling me up. This straightens my spine, brings my shoulders down and back, and opens my chest to allow for proper breathing. Always keep your knees soft (slightly bent) and your tummy tucked. Unless otherwise instructed for specific exercises, feet should be under your hips. Once you begin to grow strong this posture will come naturally and you will be standing tall and proud.

I cannot stress the importance of proper technique enough, especially when working with weights. Don't waste precious workout time pumping and straining for little or no results. Learn the proper use of the equipment and positioning of your body and watch it transform itself into something beautiful.

Maximizing Results

As you now know, it is necessary to provide your muscles with the fuel they need to perform. For maximum efficiency, eat slow burning carbohydrates, whole grain cereal or bread for instance, combined with protein, before your workout. Ideally eat or drink protein within twenty minutes of completing your workout, especially a weight-training workout. If you want to see results, following these rules will get you there faster. Of course be sure to include these calories in your daily total. To make sure I get protein to my exhausted muscles, I bring a Protein Bar or a serving of Whey Protein powder in a shaker cup. After my workout, I mix it with some water from my water bottle and drink it down. I also have a portion of fruit to complete this snack and all my nutritional needs are met. Or bring along fat free cottage cheese and fruit; however, you will have to keep it cool while you exercise. It is really quite easy once it becomes routine.

Developing good nutritional habits are essential to long-term success. According to Dr. Maxwell Maltz, it takes an average of twenty one times of completing a task to make it a habit/routine. Some people must complete the task more times and some less, but the average is twenty-one. This is really a small number. If you are exercising four or five times a week, your new routine can be established in a month. If you can stick with it that long, it will soon be part of your regular schedule, which it should be from now on.

This routine that I am talking about is the act of getting your workout done. Your workout itself should not be routine. After mastering a routine for a few weeks, change it. Try different equipment, or join a class. Switch from heavy weights to lighter weights with more repetitions, and then switch back again. Your workout should always be evolving and rotating. You will be stimulating different muscles and the same muscles in different ways. This way you will be training smaller muscle tissue as well as large. This is called *periodization*, or doing each routine for a month or so and then changing it. Your muscles have memory and once they have been trained in a particular way, they will remember that training and return to it more efficiently the more your change it up. Continually learning new routines will also keep your brain stimulated.

I have started keeping track of my workout schedule on my calendar. Even though I thought I was mixing it up regularly, when reviewing my last few months I realized I had fallen into a predictable (to my body) routine. I had been taking stationary bicycle spinning classes on Friday mornings because I liked the teacher and was learning a lot about building cardiovascular strength. One week I was unable to go on Friday, so I went on Wednesday instead. Even though I had been spinning for quite a while, my legs were screaming the next morning. It was a different instructor and a different day of the week. My body had grown accustomed to spinning on Friday with that particular instructor in a very short time. Don't let yourself be lulled into doing the same thing over and over. Your body will adapt itself and your results will diminish.

More is not always better. To get the most out of every workout don't overdo it. Doing your full cardio and weight training workouts back to back may be too much. One hour of giving it your all is a sure way of maximizing every minute of your exercise time.

To keep my workout efficient, I have learned some tricks that increase my results. Some days I work all of my upper body muscle groups with *multiple-sets* (two or three sets of 12 reps), and then spend the second half of my gym time doing the same on my lower body. Sometimes I *super-set* this workout (increasing or decreasing weights each set) for an even tougher challenge. This works the muscles to exhaustion and they will respond by increasing in strength. Another result booster is using the *antagonistic* method of working opposing muscle groups back-to-back, biceps/triceps, quadriceps/hamstring, etc. Yet another trick to increase efficiency is *circuit training*, moving quickly from one activity to the next. During circuit training you can mix cardiovascular with free weights, stationary equipment, or any activity you choose. Keep moving and you will gain some cardiovascular benefits at the same time. Additionally, alternating between upper and lower body exercises in the same workout further strengthens the heart muscle by requiring it to pump blood first to the upper body, then switch to the lower body and back again. We all want a healthy heart. The culmination of rotating these variations will result in a sharper mind, and a healthy, conditioned body, ready to take on almost anything.

Stretch and Recover

Stretching gently before you begin any physical activity is a good idea. It seems the older I get, the stiffer I am in the morning. It is not a good idea to aggressively stretch cold muscles, but a quick warm-up and some gentle stretches will warm the muscles and get the blood flowing to them. After your workout, when you are hot and sweaty, you will be able to increase your flexibility through deep, long stretches. Hold each stretch for up to twenty seconds while focusing on supplying oxygen to the muscles through smooth steady breathing. Think of creating long lean muscles while you carefully bend and reach. I consider this time my reward for completing a tough workout because it feels so good to stretch the muscles out when they are really warm. Take the time to enjoy your healthy flush and stretch it out.

By scheduling in some days off you are allowing yourself to recover. When your muscles are really sore, they are telling you to lay-off. The soreness is actually damage to the muscles, small tears that are part of the process of building stronger, healthier muscles. Given time, and proper nutrition, they will grow stronger as they heal. The improved strength will be noticeable when you resume your workouts.

You may get real sore after your first few sessions, and it is OK to take a couple of days off. As time goes by you will get less sore and one day off is sufficient. Or if you work your upper body intensely one day, rest it while you work your lower body the next. When I am working out back-to-back days, I alternate weight training with some intense cardio. I do this some of the time, but I do schedule a day or two each week to totally recover. We all have days without enough hours, and these are the perfect times to take an exercise break. It is even okay to miss a scheduled workout when life happens. Don't beat yourself up over it. Stress is a health robber and you don't want to reverse the good work you are doing. Realize that you can get back to your routine soon enough and all will be well. Remember, the picture is not complete unless your mind and spirit are nourished along with your body.

Setbacks

During the course of writing this chapter I had an equipment malfunction while skiing a steep, black diamond run at Mammoth Mountain in the southern Sierra's. I was feeling proud of my skiing ability, enjoying the scenery, great snow and the clear, cold day. Unbeknownst to me, my improperly adjusted bindings had been loosening all morning, and with no warning whatsoever, my skis flew out from under me. As I slid, rolled, bumped and banged down the mountain, I wondered how serious my injuries would be. Once the snow settled around me, the ski patrol transported me to the first aid office where the bruising and swelling began.

My broken wrist - right hand of course - and cracked ribs would need eight to ten weeks to heal and I was very concerned that I would lose all my muscle tone and gain unwanted weight. My son advised me not to worry and reassured me that since I had been in shape for so long, my body would remember my fitness level and return to it efficiently, once I resumed my workouts.

As the weeks of recovery went by, I watched my muscles gradually shrink. This distressed me until I realized that I was losing weight. Granted it was muscle tissue, but at least I was not gaining. Soon I was taking walks with neighbors and actually enjoying the change of routine. Frankly, I did not miss the gym at all.

After nine weeks I was released of all restrictions and realized I would have to practice what I am preaching in this book and begin exercising slow, eating well, and wondered if my 58-year-old body would respond like my son promised it would. I was also able to relate to you readers who are facing the challenge of beginning a fitness program. I won't tell you it was easy, but just because something is hard does not mean we shouldn't do it, right?

I was surprisingly weak when I started, and protective of my just healed bones. The good news is it took no time at all to see my muscles begin to develop and my strength increase. Within two to three months I was back to my previous fitness level and revising my vow to never ski again.

Once you get in shape, you will face setbacks of injuries, accidents, vacations, and life in general. Don't be discouraged or depressed, remember that you know how to eat right and get in shape. Our bodies really do have muscle memory and rebound pretty fast. Changing your routine – even to recover from an illness or injury – will trigger your body to respond quickly when you begin your fitness regime again.

Chapter 5

Cardiovascular for Extra Weight Loss

It Takes Work to Get That Fat Off

Now that you are becoming toned and shapely, you want to be rid of the excess baggage (fat) and show off your new physique. Some lucky people can lose weight by dieting alone, or starting an exercise program without dieting. But we post-menopausal women need to attack the enemy, unhealthy aging, from all fronts. Adding some good old fat burning cardiovascular workouts to your weight training and healthy eating program may be your key to winning the battle. In addition to burning fat, cardiovascular work will increase your stamina for physical activities and your busy everyday life. Wouldn't it be nice to still have energy late in the day? A strong heart can give you the gift of more productive hours in your day. I like to go strong all evening until my body finally puts on the brakes and signals it's time to rest. Being more active also prepares you for a better night's sleep so you wake up ready to go.

Of course you must first consider your fitness level. If you are new to exercise, start with walking or bike riding, or something manageable. Once you get comfortable, increase the time and or difficulty. Continue to increase the intensity of your workout as you grow stronger and always try to push yourself just a little past your comfort zone. Don't be afraid to sweat, it's your body's way of staying cool. Just as with your weight-training program, switching your cardiovascular routine around will prevent plateaus.

Once you become stronger you can progress to harder cardiovascular challenges. I used to peek into the spin room at the gym where exercisers were feverishly riding stationary bikes while being coached by an instructor. It looked so intense that I was afraid I would not be able to handle it. When it came time to 'switch it up', I decided to give it a try. I figured I could get a bike in the back and go at my own pace and hopefully not embarrass myself too much. I pedaled my fanny off, or almost off, and gave the ride everything I had to give. I made it to the end and even though I was physically drained, I was so proud of myself and left on an endorphin high. I stuck with it, going a couple times each week until I built up the strength and stamina to attend the class without fear. It is a killer every time I go, but what a calorie burner and endurance builder!

I have learned a lot about myself by meeting new physical challenges and digging down deep to find strength I did not think I had. Pushing just a little harder and reaching a new goal is satisfying and rewarding. When you think you have to give up, visualize trying to reach the top of a snowcapped mountain, or riding along a country road with the wind in your hair, or seeing the finish line just ahead. These images may keep you going just long enough to hit that imaginary wall. I have hit that wall on a regular basis and now know that it is very real. My favorite spin instructor encouraged me to reach my personal limit (thanks Stacy). Realize that your personal limit is unique to you and your workouts should be structured accordingly. But whatever your limit is, reach for it. When you achieve it, revel in your accomplishment.

Carol Ann Haines

Keep Your Heart Pumping

When I take time out of my busy day to exercise, I want to be sure I am getting all the benefits exercise can provide: improved stamina, physical strength, a healthy heart, and mood elevation. Knowing and monitoring your heart rate during aerobic exercise will ensure these rewards.

As we age, our heart rate gradually slows down. Therefore, your target heart rate is determined by your age. Subtracting your age from the number 226 for women and 220 for men, will give you your maximum heart rate. Use this number (mine is 168) to determine your target heart rate. If you are healthy, you should aim for a target heart rate of 50 to 80 percent of your maximum heart rate. My low end at 50 percent is 168 x .5 = 84 beats per minute (bpm), and my high end is 168 x .8 = 134 bpm. This is the range you want to be in during aerobic exercise. When you are beginning, stay in the lower range and as you become fit, the more time you spend in your high range the more intense your workout will be. If you are on heart medication, check with your doctor to see if it affects your heart rate, as your target heart rate may need to be adjusted.

The easiest way to monitor your heart rate during exercise is to use the radial pulse at the base of the thumb on either wrist, or the carotid pulse on the side of the neck. Use your index and middle finger of either hand to locate the artery and count the beats in a ten second period. To determine your bpm, multiply that number by six. If your ten-second-pulse count is 17, multiply 17 x 6, and your heart rate is 102 bpm[1].

Remember to keep your body hydrated and oxygenated before, during and after your workout. Have a water bottle with you and drink at regular intervals while you exercise. Settle into a rhythmic breathing pattern early in your workout and

---

1.   American council on exercise (ACE)

monitor that pattern throughout. Adequate water and oxygen will allow your muscles, including your heart muscle, to grow strong and healthy.

Let common sense by your guide. Listen to your body and make adjustments that work for you. Start gradually, eat right, increase intensity when you feel ready, and your workouts will be safe and effective.

Stay Motivated

Just do it. We have all seen the Nike ads exclaiming 'Just Do It'. It is a good motto to live by, especially when it comes to staying active. Instead of procrastinating and making excuses, get going and get it done, whatever 'it' is. Not doing the things we know we should do results in feelings of guilt and anxiety. Life is tough enough, why add more stress? Get your workout done and feel powerful and energized. It is a better way to approach your day, and life. This motto applies to other decisions also. A wise person once told me that when you have a decision to make, always go with the positive. When debating whether to accept an invitation, accept it. Even if you think you are too tired to go, you may end up having the time of your life, or meeting someone extraordinary. I have been following these words of wisdom for a while now, and most of the time the positive choice is the right one.

Another important reason to stick with your new healthy lifestyle is because you can. Be grateful that you can get up in the morning and go to the gym or put in an exercise DVD and workout. If you ever find yourself bedridden, you will pray for the opportunity to get out there and live. Well you have that opportunity right now, to live life to the maximum every day. Take advantage of your good health. Don't leave anything undone or end any day with regrets. Instead, drift off to sleep at night feeling fulfilled and content. We all have much to be thankful for.

Sometimes it takes another person's misfortunes to give us proper perspective of our own problems. I learned to be more grateful after recovering from another of my... incidents. I was innocently shoe shopping with girlfriends one Saturday when I spotted some really cute platform shoes. They were really high and I was not seriously considering buying them, but I thought I'd try them on to see if maybe I could actually walk in them. Well as you can probably guess it ended badly. On the first step my ankle went over the side of the shoe and it was quite a distance to the floor. The pain was intense, but I persevered through the remainder of the afternoon until I realized my foot was swelling and turning purple. Eventually, I made it to the doctor where it was confirmed that I had broken a bone in my foot. I felt like a total idiot. Who breaks their foot trying on shoes? I received an email from a friend who had heard of my dilemma which read 'News Flash! Women over forty do not wear platform shoes'. I already knew that, but I was just trying them on.

After a couple of weeks of lying around with my foot propped up, the doctor finally released me to go to the gym and ride a stationary bike, but only if I wore this funny little shoe with a wooden sole. The next day I headed out with my gym bag and wooden shoe. It rarely rains in San Diego County, but it was raining that morning and I struggled with my crutches on the slippery pavement, dropping things and feeling so sorry for myself. Why am I doing this? I should turn around and go home, I whined to myself.

Once I pushed the heavy glass door open with my backside, I hobbled past the front desk and looked around for an empty cycle. Right in front of me was a man with no legs propped up on a cycle with hand peddles just going to town on that thing. He looked like he hadn't a care in the world and was thoroughly enjoying his workout. I don't know how he even got himself up there. His smile and enthusiasm lifted my mood as I realized I had been consumed by self-pity, and it was time to buck up and start getting myself back in shape. My minor injury would be healed and forgotten in a few months. It took this contented man with a permanent disability to give me a brighter outlook as well as gratitude for my relatively good health.

Now that my foot is healed, I put it to good use whenever possible. If I can fit in a walk after dinner or take the stairs instead of an elevator, I do it, because I can. Little bursts of energy throughout the day will add up to higher daily calorie expenditure and a stronger heart.

Your twice-weekly intense cardiovascular workout, coupled with an active lifestyle including taking the stairs, choosing to walk when possible, and just keeping that body on the move, will keep your internal fire burning away that unwanted fat. Your heart will be stronger, and you will have a rosy glow in your cheeks and a sparkle in your eyes that people will be drawn to. That healthy glow is an attractive alternative to plastic surgery.

Chapter 6

Putting It All Together

Your Personal Plan

While formulating your personal fitness plan, consider your current fitness level, your daily schedule, and your likes and dislikes. I have shared my own diet and exercise plan, but make yours your own. If the plan is going to work for the long haul, it has to fit with your lifestyle. As long as you include the four keys: positive attitude, calorie conscience diet, weight training, and cardiovascular exercise, you can't go wrong. If you are a non-exerciser, start slow. A ten-minute walk around the neighborhood, and some repetitions with one or two pound dumb-bells may be your starting place. Remember, any exercise is better than none. Gradually increasing the duration and intensity of your workout will increase your strength and stamina. Practice body awareness as you begin and don't overdo it. Listen to your body as it tells you when to back off and when it can do more.

When I started my program so long ago, my trainer instructed me to stay off the scale for six weeks. I did not know if I would be able to do it, but I did. What made staying off the scale easy was the fact that very soon after starting my diet and exercise routines my clothes began to get loose. By the time six weeks had passed I could not wear any of my pants without them falling down. When I finally weighed myself, I was happy to see I had lost pounds, but happier yet that I had lost a size or two.

The reason for not weighing in the early weeks of your program is that you will be gaining muscle. Muscle, being denser than voluminous fat, weighs more. You may actually gain weight even though your clothes are getting loose. It would be discouraging to weigh after the first weeks of dedication and not see any results on the scale. Instead, marvel at your baggie pants and too big blouses and let your body reshape itself before you start weighing yourself.

Once you are ready to start weighing in, plan to do it once a week. Try to weigh at the same time of day as your weight fluctuates (increases) throughout the day. Some people weigh every day, but most of us post-menopausal women will have fluctuations due to water retention caused by a number of elements, so we may get discouraged by weighing every day. Try once a week and each time you should see a loss and be motivated and proud. Don't expect large, sudden weight reductions. A slow steady weight loss will be a more permanent loss.

Prepare

I love organization. I am a list maker, plan follower, and I get satisfaction from checking accomplished tasks off my numerous lists. You may not be a fanatic like me, but I do recommend making preparations before you start. If you are not a list maker, I happen to have one right here.

1.   Get mentally prepared.
       a. Make up your mind to follow your plan and feel good about your decision to get lean and strong.

2. Plan your diet.
   a. Clear your kitchen and workspace of unhealthy, high calorie, tempting food.
   b. Assemble light, healthy recipes (I have included some of my favorites).
   c. Make menus for the upcoming week.
   d. Shop and stock your refrigerator and pantry with lots of healthy foods. Purchase everything you will need for meals and snacks to get you started. Include staples that should always be in your pantry (see list).
   e. Purchase a food scale with ounces and grams.
   f. Purchase an insulated lunch bag with freezer packs for on the go meals and snacks.
3. Get ready to exercise.
   a. Decide when and where you will work out (a weekly exercise plan works for me). Join a gym, hire a trainer, or find DVDs for home use. Whichever route you are taking, get prepared. Remember to include both cardiovascular and weight training workouts each week.
   b. Purchase good shoes and active wear. Don't buy too much as you may need smaller sizes in the near future.
   c. Get your starting weight and measurements.
   d. Take a before picture.
   e. If you have any health concerns talk to your doctor so you can begin with confidence.

Once everything on the list is checked off you are ready to start your personal fitness plan. Look forward to being and looking better with each new day from now on. You should be feeling empowered right now. These changes you are making in your routine are all positive and rewarding changes. I am excited for you!

Success Stories

To help you understand how plans can vary, I am including some success stories. These stories are from real women in their late fifties who have conquered the post-menopausal weight gain and energy drain. They look and live like women much younger than they are.

Peggy

Like so many of us Peggy has watched her weight all her life. She has been on every diet that came along and was able to manage her weight well enough until her late forties. Combined with perimenopause and a stressful new full time job, she began to gain and soon realized she was twenty-five pounds overweight.

Peggy had dreamed of owning a horse for four decades. During this complicated time she was able to fulfill that dream and began to ride on a regular basis. One of her riding companions happened to be Loren, a six foot tall, slender and shapely, Belgian model. Then the fateful day arrived when she saw a picture of herself on her horse and mentally compared that picture to the way Loran looked on her horse. The comparison was the inspiration Peggy needed to get back in shape. After so many years of longing for a horse, she wanted to look good when she rode it, and resolved to make it happen.

Horseback riding is the core of Peggy's fitness routine. She has become a dedicated rider and rides two or three times each week. How perfect is that? To be passionate about your workout is a key to success. In addition to riding she takes stairs instead of elevators, chooses to park further back in parking lots, and takes walks when time permits.

For diet management Peggy chose the tried and true method of calorie counting. She determined how many calories were needed for a healthy weight loss program and wrote down everything she ate. Eight months later she was twenty-five pounds lighter and looking fantastic on that horse. She lost approximately three pounds a month, which is a healthy (and much more likely to be permanent) rate of weight loss.

At fifty-nine Peggy is full of life and likes to shop for bargains on designer jeans that fit snug and look amazing on her. She now knows how to eat properly and if those jeans get a little too tight, she goes back to counting calories until they fit properly again. Happy trails to you Peggy!

Rita

Rita is my beautiful lifelong friend with the Mediterranean skin that doesn't wrinkle, the striking dark features ala Sophia Loren, and a recently trimmed and toned body. Her parents are Italian and around her childhood home, homemade pastas, sauces, breads, meats and cheeses were commonplace. Consequently, Rita carried a little extra weight for most of her life. Like me, by her fifties she was about twenty pounds overweight. Over the years she, like a lot of us, tried every fad diet that came along. She would lose the weight, but sadly, always regained it.

One of Rita's daughters, being brought up with the same great homemade Italian foods, also struggled with her weight. Together they decided to join Weight Watchers and adopt a healthier lifestyle. This venture marked the end of Rita's fad dieting. At Weight Watchers she learned to forget that disheartening word 'diet' and to focus on eating the foods that keep her energized and lean. Although she has a full time job, she is a dedicated exerciser, including a few trips to the gym each week, swimming, walking, or whatever activity fits into her busy schedule.

Rita lost that unwanted twenty pounds and now looks and feels fabulous. Her keys to success include realizing that fitness is a lifelong commitment, not a diet. She recommends when choosing your exercise program, do what you like. If you enjoy it, you are much more likely to stay motivated. Lean meats, whole grains, fresh fruits and vegetables comprise most of her healthy diet.

Managing stress plays an important role in Rita's program as well. Balancing work, aging parents, children, and social commitments can overwhelm the most organized among us. When stress threatens to upset Rita's apple cart, she puts the brakes on for a little while. Finding time to rest her mind is as important as the other elements of her fitness routine. Spending a little quiet time with her thoughts freshens her perspective and gives her the strength to manage her sometimes-hectic life.

Diane

Diane put on weight during high school. In her late teens she went to Germany as an exchange student and the weight came off. She attributes this to the German tradition of eating the main meal at noon and eating light for dinner. Unfortunately she returned home to emotional upheaval and regained what she had lost.

As an impressionable young woman she latched onto whatever diet was popular at the moment and began jogging on the beach and doing yoga. When the current diet became impossible to maintain, she would switch to another one, and the weight loss, regain, cycle began.

As time went by Diane realized this yo-yo dieting and regaining was not working. These restrictive diets where not maintainable and were shutting down her metabolism. She resolved to begin eating a healthy, low calorie diet, and you should see her now!

Diane's life continues to challenge her, with the loss of her beautiful home in the 2007 San Diego wild fires and the breakup of her marriage soon after. Today she is the mother of two teenagers and working to build a new life as a single woman. Through it all she has continued to eat well and never misses her daily workout or an opportunity to ride her horse. She rises at 4:30am, puts in an exercise DVD, and gets it done. For me this routine is a little intense, as I need my sleep and a day or two free of workouts. However, Diane looks spectacular! There is not an ounce of excess fat on that woman. When she wears a tank top, all you see are lean, sculpted shoulders and arms. No unsightly bulges around the bra line on that body.

For Diane, healthy eating and dedication to exercise has kept her grounded through some tough times, as well as keeping her looking fantastic.

These women inspire and encourage me. They are beyond beautiful, full of energy, quick witted, and fun to be around. I am lucky to have such exceptional women in my life. They have taken control of their physical and emotional lives, and so can you.

Mark's Success Story

I am including my husband Mark's story even though he is not a post-menopausal woman. As I have mentioned, this program works for everyone. His story demonstrates the importance of nourishing your body sufficiently during your fitness transformation. Mark's story began when he was 55 years old, 25-30 pounds overweight, and outgrowing his 'fat clothes'. Like Peggy, his wake up call came when he saw a photo of himself in bathing trunks and realized it was time to make a change.

Mark had a history of back pain and old injuries, so our son, Ryan, being inexperienced at training people with injuries, set him up with a trainer he thought would be more suitable for his dad. Mark's starting weight was 190 pounds with a body mass index of 28% fat. He was to work with his trainer three times a week, add a few workouts on his own, and stick to a 1750-calorie diet (we did not know at the time that this was not enough calories).

My husband committed to the program with a vengeance. He worked out almost every day and weighed all his food, staying at or below the 1750 calories. After six months he had dropped the 30 pounds.

In the meantime Ryan, our son, was becoming more educated and experienced. He dropped by one June afternoon and caught Mark out by the pool in his bathing suit. He was shocked at Mark's appearance and exclaimed, "You are not losing unwanted weight, you are wasting away".

Ryan took Mark on as his own client and upon further evaluation they realized that although Mark had lost 30 pounds, he had only lost 1% of his body fat. The previous trainer had not monitored Mark's progress properly and the result of too few calories was a drastic loss of muscle and very little fat loss. He had been training his body to hold on to his fat stores. He did not look good and one friend commented that he looked peaked and old. Mark was very disheartened after being so dedicated only to discover he had not lost fat, but muscle, which we want for strength and vigor.

Ryan bought Mark a 'Body Bug' for father's day which he wore on his upper arm to monitor his calorie expenditure each day so they would know more accurately how many calories he needed. With Mark's dedication to working out, he was burning between 2600 and 2800 calories a day. Ryan's guidelines for healthy weight loss require the dieter to stay at or below a 500-calorie deficit. He increased Mark's calories to 2250 a day.

After six weeks of working with Ryan it was time to evaluate Mark's progress. His weight was the same but his body fat was down to 22%. He had lost fat and gained muscle. His measurements increased in the right places (biceps and chest) and decreased around the waist. In this short time he lost that sickly look and was beginning to look healthy, fit and trim. What a difference an increase in calories made.

Five years later Mark continues to eat six times a day and exercise regularly. He looks great for a 60-year old and is the only man I know in his age group that does not take any medication. His blood pressure and cholesterol numbers are perfect. His experience with eating too few calories demonstrated to us the importance of eating enough. To lose the fat, you have to feed the muscles or you will lose them first. Get all the calories you need to grow strong and lean!

Chapter 7

Meal Plans, Recipes and Snack Ideas

Meal Plans

Eating healthy is not that complicated. Think fresh, whole, natural and lean. Roasting, grilling, and steaming are easier cooking methods than frying. Fresh herbs and spices accent the flavor of foods without adding fat and calories. So what did my weight loss diet look like? Here are a few samples (calories are approximate).

Sample Menu 1

300-calorie Breakfast	Oatmeal, ½ grapefruit, ½ cup of soymilk divided between oatmeal and coffee, and 1/3 serving of whey protein
150-calorie snack	Light yogurt and 1 serving of fruit
300-calorie lunch	Salad with 2-3 cups mixed greens and vegetables, 1 tablespoon of nuts, 1 tablespoon of

goat cheese and 3oz of chicken or other lean protein, Light dressing. Herbal tea or water

150-calorie snack	One hundred calorie popped corn and 1 serving of fruit
450-calorie dinner	4oz poultry, fish, lean meat or pork, 1 medium redskin potato baked with skin, sprayed with 'I Can't Believe It's Not Butter", and lots of vegetables
150-calorie snack	½ cup fat free cottage cheese and fruit

Sample Menu 2

300-calorie breakfast	Egg substitute (Egg Beaters) omelet - (3 servings Egg Beaters), 2 oz. low fat cheddar cheese. Add a few mushrooms, onions, or 1 T. salsa to taste. ½ cup halved strawberries, ½ whole-wheat English muffin
150-calorie snack	2 rice cakes, 1 T. peanut butter
300-calorie lunch	Turkey sandwich (2 slices light bread, 4 oz turkey breast, mustard, lettuce, tomato), 1 med. apple
150-calorie snack	1 oz whole-grain tortilla chips, 2 T. fresh salsa

450-calorie dinner	See menu 1. Substitute potato with whole-grain rice or whole-wheat roll and use your imagination, just watch your calories and don't forget your veggies
150-calorie snack	100 calories Wheat Thins pack and 1 wedge light Laughing Cow cheese

Sample Menu 3

300-calorie breakfast	1 cup of whole grain cereal, 1 cup skim milk, 1 small banana
150-calorie snack	1 serving protein powder, 1 serving fruit
300-calorie lunch	4 oz grilled shrimp, 2 cups green salad with 2 T light dressing and 1 small whole wheat roll
150-calorie snack	½ oz almonds and 1 oz raisins
450-calorie dinner	2 oz whole grain thin spaghetti, 1 ½ cup Prego or other sauce, 2 T parmesan cheese, 1 small whole grain roll, veggies
150-calorie snack	¾ cup slow churned ice cream

These menus total approximately 1500 calories per day. Of course these menus varied from day to day, but the calories remained the same. Now that I have reached my goal weight, my daily caloric intake can increase up to about 2000. This extra 500 calories gives me plenty of leeway to keep the weight off, which I have done for five years. This is a workable plan. Find that mental place you need to be at to make the commitment and just do it!

Pantry Staples - Things I Always Have on Hand

Whole Grain Rice
Oatmeal and other Whole Grain Cereal
Whole Grain Pasta
Unsalted Nuts
Light Salad Dressings
Frozen and Canned Vegetables
Stevia Artificial Sweetener
Olive Oil and Olive Oil Spray
Honey
Mustard
Vinegar (Red Wine, Cider, etc.)
Light Jam
Rice Cakes
Potatoes and Sweet Potatoes
100 Calorie Popped Corn
I Can't Believe its Not Butter Spray
Raisins
Sesame and Sun Flower Seeds
Whey Protein Powder
Protein Bars
Peanut Butter

Weekly Shopping Regulars

Fat Free Milk or Soy/Almond Milk
Lean Poultry, Fish, Meat, or Pork
Light or Fat Free Yogurt
Fat Free Cottage Cheese
Goat Cheese or Feta Crumbles
Eggs and Egg Whites
Light or Fat Free Sour Cream
Whole Grain Bread/English Muffins (Sara Lee
    Delightful at 45 Cals per slice is my favorite)
Variety of Fresh Fruits
Variety of Fresh Vegetable
Fresh Salsa
Laughing Cow Light Cheese Wedges

150-Calorie Snack Ideas

½ Cup Fat Free Cottage Cheese with Veggie Sticks
  or Fruit

Yogurt with Fruit

1oz Whole Grain Corn Chips with 2 Tablespoons
  Fresh Salsa

2 Rice Cakes with 2 Wedges of Light Laughing
  Cow Cheese

2 Rice Cakes with 1 Tablespoon Peanut Butter

1 Whole Wheat English Muffin with 2 Tablespoons
  of Light Jam

1 Dozen Almonds with 2 Tablespoons of Raisins

1 Slice of Whole Grain Toast with 1 Tablespoon
  of Peanut Butter

1 Small Apple with 1 Tablespoon of Peanut Butter

100 Calorie Popped Corn and 1 Serving of Fruit

Hard Boiled Egg with 1 Serving of Fruit or Vegetables

Smoothie (See Recipe)

Whey Protein Powder Mixed with Water

Protein Bar (check calories)

2/3 Cup Cereal (Cheerios, etc.) and ½ Cup of Fat
  Free Milk

And for a treat, Slow Churned Ice cream

These are just a few ideas to get you started. You can eat anything that has nutritional value, as long as you limit the calories. Happy Snacking!

RECIPES

I am including several chicken recipes, as chicken is light, inexpensive, and always available. It can be prepared in a variety of ways that will please even the most discriminating of palates. The recipes have been collected from friends, Eating Light Magazine, Weight Watchers and other publications. I am sure you have some of your own and will collect more over time.

I have included only a few beef, pork, and seafood recipes even though I do eat all of these foods. When I eat them though, they are usually grilled with a little olive oil and seasonings. No recipe needed. Living in San Diego County gives me access to lots of fresh seafood, which I like grilled with fresh lemon or limejuice.

CHICKEN

PEAR/CRANBERRY CHICKEN
(217 Calories per cup)
4 servings

12oz boneless, skinless chicken breast cut into 1-inch pieces
1½ tablespoon flour
½ teaspoon salt
½ teaspoon pepper
2 teaspoons canola oil
1 ripe pear, peeled, pared and chopped
3 sliced scallions (green onion)
¾ cup pear nectar
¼ cup dried cranberries
2 teaspoons coarse grain mustard (Dijon)

1. Combine flour and ¼ teaspoon of both salt and pepper in large zip-lock baggie. Add chicken and shake to coat.

2. Heat 1 ½ teaspoons oil in large skillet and add chicken. Brown about 4-5 minutes. Put chicken on plate.

3. Add rest of oil, pear, and scallions to pan and cook on medium high heat (3 minutes) until pear is golden. Add pear nectar, cranberries and rest of salt and pepper. Increase heat to high to thicken (about 3 minutes). Add mustard and chicken and heat through.

4. Serve with whole grain brown or wild rice and vegetables.

This is one of my favorites. It is relatively easy and really delicious!

CHICKEN WITH APPLES AND CIDER
(352 Calories per serving)
4 Servings

2 tablespoons vegetable oil
1 Granny Smith apple, cored and sliced
1 tablespoon packed dark brown sugar
4-4 ounce skinless boneless chicken breasts
¼ teaspoon cinnamon
¼ teaspoon salt
¼ teaspoon freshly ground pepper
1 medium onion, thinly sliced and separated into rings
½ cup apple cider
¼ cup cider vinegar
2 cups hot cooked wide noodles

1. In a large nonstick skillet over medium heat, heat 1 tablespoon of the oil. Sauté the apple until lightly browned, about 5 minutes. Sprinkle with the brown sugar; stirring frequently, until tender, 4-5 minutes longer. Place on plate.

2. On a sheet of wax paper, sprinkle the chicken with cinnamon, salt, and pepper. In the skillet, heat the remaining 1-tablespoon oil. Sauté the chicken until browned, about 4-5 minutes on each side. Transfer to another plate.

3. In the skillet, cook the onion, covered, until tender, 7-8 minutes; stir in the cider and vinegar. Reduce the heat and simmer 2-3 minutes. Return the chicken to the skillet; simmer, spooning the sauce over chicken, until

chicken is cooked through and liquid is reduced by half, 3-5 minutes.

4.   Return the apples to the skillet; cook until heated through, (2 minutes). Arrange the noodles on a platter; top with chicken mixture, pouring any remaining juices over chicken.

5.   The sweet apples and savory onions combine in a burst of flavor. Add some vegetables and you have a great meal.

WILD MUSHROOM AND GOAT CHEESE-STUFFED CHICKEN BREAST
(252 Calories per serving) 4 Servings

3 teaspoons extra-virgin olive oil
2 garlic cloves, minced
½ pound fresh shiitake mushrooms, stems removed and caps finely chopped
¾ teaspoon Herbes de Provence
¾ teaspoon salt
¼ teaspoon freshly ground pepper
2 ounces reduced-fat goat cheese, softened
4 ¼ pounds skinless, boneless, chicken-breast halves
1 shallot, chopped
¾ cup reduced-sodium chicken broth
6 tablespoons dry sherry or orange juice
1 teaspoons cornstarch
2 teaspoons cold water

1.   To make the filling, heat 2 teaspoons of the oil in a large nonstick skillet over medium-high heat. Add the garlic and cook until fragrant, about 30 seconds. Add the mushrooms, Herbes de Povence, ¼ teaspoon of the salt, and 1/8 teaspoon of the pepper, cook, stirring occasionally, until the mushrooms are golden, about 5-6 minutes. Transfer the mixture to a bowl; add the cheese and stir until combined. Cool completely.

2.   Make a pocket in the side of each chicken breast by inserting a sharp paring knife into the thickest part and gently cutting back and forth until a small chamber opens in the side. Do not cut through to the back or side of breast. Enlarge the pockets gently with your fingers. Stuff each with 2 tablespoons of the filling.

3.   Wipe out the skillet with paper towels. Add the
        remaining 1-teaspoon oil and heat over medium heat.
        Add the chicken and sprinkle with the remaining ½
        teaspoon salt and 1/8 teaspoon pepper. Cook until the
        chicken is browned on the outside and cooked through,
        about 7-8 minutes on each side. Cut each breast into 4
        or 5 slices, transfer to a serving plate, and keep warm.

4.   To make the sauce, add the shallot to the skillet and
        cook until fragrant (30 seconds). Add the broth and
        sherry, bring to a boil. Reduce the heat and simmer 3
        minutes. Meanwhile, dissolve the cornstarch in the cold
        water in a small bowl. Stir the cornstarch mixture into
        the skillet and cook, stirring constantly, until the
        mixture bubbles and thickens (1 minute). Pour the
        sauce over the chicken before serving.

        This one requires more effort, but it is impressive when
you want a special meal.

ORANGE-CRUMBED BAKED CHICKEN
(179 Calories per serving)
4 Servings

2 tablespoons orange juice
2 tablespoons Dijon mustard
¼ teaspoon salt
¾ cup whole-wheat cracker crumbs
1 tablespoon grated orange zest
1 shallot, finely chopped
¼ teaspoon freshly ground pepper
4 (3-ounce) skinless boneless chicken thighs

1. Preheat the oven to 350 degrees; spray a nonstick baking sheet with nonstick cooking spray.

2. In a small bowl, combine the orange juice, mustard, and salt. On a sheet of wax paper, combine the cracker crumbs, orange zest, shallot, and pepper. Brush the chicken on both sides with the mustard mixture, then dredge in the crumbs, firmly pressing the crumbs to coat both sides. Place the chicken on the baking sheet. Bake about 15 minutes; turn over and bake until cooked through, 15-20 minutes longer.

The orange and shallot flavors give this dish a unique twist.

CHICKEN PARMIGIANA
(210 Calories per serving)
4 Servings

1 large egg
1-tablespoon water
½ cup plain dried bread crumbs
¼ cup chopped flat-leaf parsley
3-tablespoons freshly grated Parmesan cheese
Freshly ground pepper to taste
4 (1/4-pound) skinless, boneless chicken breast, pounded thin

1. Preheat the oven to 400 degrees. Spray a 1-quart shallow baking dish with nonstick spray.

2. Beat the egg with the water in a shallow bowl. Combine the breadcrumbs, parsley, cheese, and pepper on a sheet of wax paper.

3. Dip the chicken breasts first in the egg mixture, then coat lightly on both sides with the bread crumb mixture, shaking off the excess, and place them in the baking dish. (Discard any leftover egg or bread crumb mixture). Bake until cooked through, golden and crisp-edged (15 minutes).

Serve this with a little whole grain pasta and a light marinara sauce. As always, lots of grilled or roasted vegetables.

NANCY'S GRILLED CHICKEN
(125 Calories per serving)
4 Servings

4 tablespoons white wine or cider vinegar
1-tablespoon olive oil
1-teaspoon balsamic vinegar
1 garlic clove, minced
1 tablespoon Santa Maria Seasoning Mix (or herbs and seasonings of your choice)
4 (4 ounce) boneless, skinless, chicken breasts

1.   Mix all ingredients except chicken.

2.   Place chicken in large zip-lock baggie.

3.   Pour marinade/rub in bag and rub into chicken.

4.   Refrigerate for up to 24 hours.

5.   Grill and enjoy.

This is a summer-time favorite served with lots of grilled vegetables.

GREEK TOMATO-FETA CHICKEN CUTLETS
(163 Calories per serving)
4 Servings

4 (3 ounce) thin sliced chicken breast cutlets
1 teaspoon dried oregano
½ teaspoon salt
½ teaspoon freshly ground pepper
1 ½ teaspoons olive oil
1-pint cherry tomatoes
1 garlic clove, minced
½ teaspoon grated lemon zest
½ cup diced cucumber
¼ cup crumbled reduced-fat feta cheese
¼ cup chopped fresh mint

1.   Sprinkle the chicken with the oregano and ¼ teaspoon each of the salt and pepper. Heat 1 teaspoon of the oil in a large nonstick skillet over medium-high heat. Add the chicken and cook until browned and cooked through, around 2 minutes on each side. Transfer the chicken to a serving plate, cover and keep warm.

2.   Add the remaining ½ teaspoon oil to the same skillet, then add the tomatoes, garlic, lemon zest, and the remaining ¼ teaspoon of salt and pepper. Cook over medium-high heat, stirring often, until the tomatoes soften and collapse (3 minutes).

3.   Spoon the sauce over the chicken then sprinkle with the cucumber, cheese, and mint.

Warm pita bread goes well with this.

SALSA CHICKEN
(247 Calories per serving)
6 Servings

1-pound skinless, boneless chicken breast (I use tenders)
1 (16-ounce) jar of salsa (La Victoria, Picante, etc.). I use mild
1 (15-ounce) can of black beans
1 (15-ounce) can of corn, drained
1 (8-ounce) fat free or light cream cheese

1. Cut chicken breasts into smaller pieces (4 per breast) or use tenders.

2. Place chicken, salsa, black beans and corn in large pot or crock-pot.

3. Cook on low for 5 – 6 hours. (If using crock-pot can cook longer on low).

4. ½ hour before serving, add the cream cheese and continue cooking until the cream cheese melts (about 30 minutes).

This is easy to put in the crock-pot before you head out the door in the morning. It is good with rice and a salad.

PORK

When you buy pork always choose the loin cuts, loin chops, pork loin roast, etc. The loin is the leanest cut and really not much higher in calories than chicken. A 40-gram loin pork chop is about 100 calories. The secret is to not overcook these lean cuts or they will be dry and tough.

HONEY-MUSTARD PORK CHOPS
(178 Calories per serving)
4 Servings

4 teaspoons honey
½ cup Dijon mustard
1 teaspoon cider or white-wine vinegar
¼ teaspoon salt
Fresh ground pepper to taste
4 (5-ounce) bone-in loin pork chops, 1-inch thick

1. To prepare the marinade, liquefy the honey (I microwave it for a few seconds). Stir in mustard, vinegar, salt, and pepper; cool to room temperature.

2. Place the pork chops in a gallon-size zip-close plastic bag, add the marinade. Seal the bag, squeezing out the air, turn to coat the chops.

3. Refrigerate, turning the bag occasionally, at least 8 hours or overnight.

4. Remove the chops from the refrigerator about 30 minutes before broiling.

5.   Preheat the broiler. Discard the marinade. Broil 3-4 inches from the heat until cooked through, 6-7 minutes on each side.

This is really tasty, and easy! Just remember to get the chops in the marinade in the morning or the day before, like I do.

OVEN-BARBECUED PORK ROAST
(217 Calories per serving)
6 Servings

1 ½ pound pork loin roast
2 red delicious apples, peeled, cored and chopped
1-cup fresh or frozen cranberries
¼ cup barbecue sauce
2 tablespoons firmly packed light brown sugar

1.   Preheat oven to 325 degrees F.

2.   Place the pork on a rack in a shallow roasting pan. Roast until the pork is browned and the center reaches 165 degrees F on a meat thermometer, around 1 hour and 20 minutes.

3.   Meanwhile, in a medium saucepan, combine the apples, cranberries, barbecue sauce, sugar and ¼ cup water; bring to a boil. Reduce the heat and simmer, uncovered, stirring as needed, until the cranberries pop and the sauce is slightly thickened (15 minutes). Place the pork on a serving platter and slice. Spoon the sauce over the pork slices.

For a quick and easy sauce to serve with a pork loin roast, mix 1 part Chili Sauce with 1 part light or sugar-free jam (I like boysenberry). Heat in microwave for a few seconds and presto, you have a sauce to serve with your roast.

MAPLE-SOY GLAZED PORK CHOPS
(135 Calories per serving)
4 Servings

2 tablespoons maple syrup
2 tablespoons soy sauce
¼ teaspoon crushed red pepper
4 boneless pork loin chops

1.   Whisk first three ingredients together in a bowl, and set aside. Preheat a nonstick skillet, coat with cooking spray.

2.   Sear the chops about three minutes per side or until done. Remove from pan.

3.   Brush one tablespoon of mixture on each chop, and serve.

This can be prepared in a few minutes. Remember to cook the chops **just** until done so they are not dry.

MORE GREAT RECIPES

SHRIMP DIAVOLO
(367 Calories per serving)
4 Servings

1 pound large shrimp, peeled and deveined
3/4-teaspoon salt
4 teaspoons extra-virgin olive oil
2 garlic cloves, minced
1 teaspoon dried oregano
¼ teaspoon crushed red pepper
1 (15-ounce) can crushed tomatoes
3 tablespoons tomato paste
½ pound whole-wheat linguine or spaghetti

1.	Sprinkle the shrimp with ½ teaspoon of the salt. Heat 2 teaspoons of the oil in a large nonstick skillet over medium-high heat. Add half the shrimp and cook until golden and just opaque in the center, about 2 minutes on each side. Transfer the shrimp to a plate with a slotted spoon. Repeat with the remaining shrimp.

2.	Heat the remaining 2 teaspoons oil in the same skillet over medium heat. Add the garlic, oregano, and crushed red pepper; cook, stirring constantly, until fragrant, about 30 seconds. Stir in the tomatoes and tomato paste; cook until slightly thickened, 5-6 minutes. Add the shrimp and the remaining ¼ teaspoon salt; cook, stirring occasionally, until heated through, about 1 minute.

3.   Meanwhile, cook the linguine according to package
      directions; drain in a colander. Divide the linguine
      among 4 plates, and top each serving with the sauce.

      If crushed red pepper is too much for your taste buds,
omit it, or cut it to 1/8 teaspoon. Enjoy!

TACO SOUP
(190 Calories per serving)
6-8 (10-Ounce) Servings

1 pound lean ground turkey
1 onion, chopped
4 cans Mexican style tomatoes
1 can kidney beans
1 can black beans
1 can corn
1 small can sliced olives
1 package taco seasoning

1.   Brown turkey and onion in large soup pot.

2.   Add rest of ingredients, stir, heat through and serve.
      The longer it simmers the better it gets. I make it in the
      morning and simmer it all day.

3.   Top with a dollop of fat free or light sour cream and
      crumbled tortilla chips.

This is a regular at my house. I like to have the
leftovers in the refrigerator for quick lunches or dinners. It's
even better the second or third day.

BUTTERNUT SQASH SOUP
(114 Calories per serving)
6 Servings

2 tablespoons butter
½ cup chopped onions
Pinch nutmeg
1Golden Delicious apple, peeled, cored and diced
2 teaspoon grated fresh ginger
6 cups nonfat chicken broth
1 small butternut squash, peeled, halved, seeded and cut into
 bite-size pieces*
salt and pepper to taste

1.   In a medium stockpot, combine butter, onions, nutmeg
       and apple pieces. Cook on medium for about 5 minutes.
       Add ginger, broth and squash and bring to a boil.
       Reduce heat and simmer, uncovered, for 25 minutes.
       Stir in salt and pepper.

2.   Working in batches, let soup cool slightly, then
       puree in a blender until smooth.

3.   Return pureed soup to cooking pot and bring to
       simmer. Serve with a dab of low-fat sour cream and
       fresh herbs.

       *Use a potato peeler to peel the squash. To soften
       enough to cut, microwave large pieces for about 40
       seconds.

       This creamy, sweet soup will warm you on a crisp
autumn day.

VEGETABLES

Vegetables should be front and center when planning your healthy diet. They should be a large part of all your meals, except breakfast, which is a great time to eat fruit. Do your best to eat fresh and organic and include some raw vegetables every day. A large lunch salad is light and refreshing, or a side salad at dinner. Grab carrots, celery, radishes, sliced bell peppers, and cucumbers for easy snacks. I like grilled and roasted vegetables in addition to fresh. Steaming is another healthy option. Try some of the recipes below and find out how delicious veggies can be.

FAVORITE LIGHT SALAD DRESSINGS AND MARINADES

Brianna's Special Request Lemon Tarragon, 35 calories per 2 tablespoon serving

Brianna's Special Request Santa Fe Blend, 25 calories per 2 tablespoon serving

Newman's Own Light Balsamic, 45 Calories per 2 tablespoon serving

Bernstein's Light Cheese Fantastico, 25 calories per 2 tablespoon serving

Kraft Roasted Red Pepper Italian with Parmesan, 40 calories per 2 tablespoon serving.

BASIC GRILLING OR ROASTING VEGETABLES

Bell pepper	Carrots
Onion	Cauliflower
Asparagus	Eggplant
Cherry tomatoes	Parsnip
Potatoes	Rutabaga
Sweet potatoes	Winter squash
Mushrooms	Zucchini
Broccoli	Crookneck squash
Beets	

Cut any of the veggies listed (or any of your own choosing) into large pieces

Toss with 1 tablespoon of olive oil and seasonings of choice

For roasting, spread out on a jellyroll or pizza pan and roast at 400 degrees F for 20 to 30 minutes, stirring halfway through cooking.

For grilling, place in a vented, sided, barbecue-grilling pan. Grill on medium heat for 15 to 20 minutes, stirring frequently.

LEMON-CHIVE ROASTED VEGETABLES
(129 Calories per serving)
6 servings

3/4 pound small red potatoes, halved
3/4 pound small fingerling potatoes, halved
1/2 pound baby carrots
1 medium Vidalia or other sweet onion, cut into 8 wedges
1/2-tablespoon olive oil
Cooking spray
1 tablespoon chopped fresh chives
3/4 teaspoons grated lemon rind
1 tablespoon fresh lemon juice
1/4-teaspoon salt
1/8-teaspoon black pepper

1.   Preheat oven to 425 degrees F.

2.   Combine first 5 ingredients in a large bowl; toss well to
        coat. Arrange vegetables in a single layer on a jellyroll
        pan coated with cooking spray. Bake at 425 degrees F
        for 30 minutes, turning after about 15 minutes or until
        tender and lightly browned.

3.   Combine vegetables, chives and remaining ingredients
        in a large bowl; Toss gently to coat.

        This recipe dresses your roasted veggies up a little bit.

BAKED CROOKNECK SQUASH AND TOMATOES
(77 Calories per serving)
8 servings

4 medium (200 gram) crookneck squash, sliced
4 medium tomatoes, sliced
2 green onions, chopped
2 tablespoons red wine vinegar
2 tablespoons olive oil
1 tablespoon Dijon mustard
½ teaspoon salt
½ teaspoon freshly ground black pepper

1. Preheat oven to 400 degrees F. Lightly grease a 1 quart casserole dish.

2. Alternate slices of the squash and tomatoes in the prepared casserole dish, and sprinkle with green onions. Mix the vinegar, oil, mustard, salt, and pepper in a bowl, and drizzle over the vegetables.

3. Bake 15 or 20 minutes in the preheated oven, or until squash is tender. Cool around 15 minutes before serving.

I fix this all summer when we have fresh tomatoes and squash from our garden. It is a really good blend of flavors. When we have lots of fresh vegetables, I double the recipe and bake it in an 8 x 11 baking dish so we have leftovers.

BAKED SWEET POTATO FRIES
(166 Calories per serving)
4 – 6 servings

4 sweet potatoes
¼ cup olive oil
Salt to taste

1.   Preheat oven to 400 degrees F.

2.   Cut sweet potatoes into about ½-inch thick lengthwise
        strips and toss with olive oil.

3.   Coat a baking sheet with nonstick cooking spray and
        arrange potatoes on baking sheet.

4.   Bake potatoes for 15 to 20 minutes or until golden
        brown on bottom. Turn potatoes over and bake another
        15 to 20 minutes or until golden brown all over.
        Sprinkle with salt and serve

This is a great side dish and really satisfying.

CUCUMBER-DILL SALAD
(38 Calories per serving)
4 Servings

2   cucumbers
1   tablespoon cider or white vinegar
2   teaspoons of sugar
1   teaspoon salt and freshly ground pepper to taste
1   small red onion, sliced and broken into rings
3   tablespoons finely chopped fresh dill

Thinly slice the cucumber widthwise. Place the vinegar, sugar, salt, and pepper in a bowl and whisk until the sugar is dissolved. Add the cucumber, onion and dill, and toss well. The salad can be served at once, but to improve in flavor, let the ingredients marinate.

Cucumber and dill go so well together. Another summer favorite

GRAPEFRUIT AND AVOCADO SALAD
(269 Calories per serving)
4 Servings

1-bag spring-mix greens
2 tablespoons red-wine vinegar
2 tablespoons olive oil
Juice and grated zest from 1 orange
Salt and pepper, to taste
1 red grapefruit, peeled, trimmed of white membranes and cut into pieces
2 avocados, peeled and sliced
2 tablespoons toasted pine nuts

Rinse greens and pat dry. Place in a large bowl and set aside. In a small bowl, whisk together vinegar, olive oil, orange juice, orange zest, salt and pepper. Toss the greens with two-thirds of the dressing. Divide greens among four serving plates. Top with grapefruit and avocado and drizzle with remaining dressing. Sprinkle with toasted pine nuts.

If you love red grapefruit like I do, you will love this salad!

FRUIT SMOOTHIE
(160 Calories per serving)
1 Serving

½ banana
½ cup fresh or frozen berries (any fruit will work)
¼ serving of vanilla Whey Protein Powder
¼ cup yogurt
splash of fruit juice
sweetener to taste
2/3 cup crushed ice

Put all ingredients in blender and blend until smooth. Yummy!!

If you don't have protein powder or plain yogurt, I have used fat-free cottage cheese for the protein, and it worked well. However, I like the tang the yogurt adds. Great summertime snack!

VIRTUOUS CHEESECAKE
(147 Calories per serving)
8 Servings

2 (8-ounce) containers nonfat cream cheese
½ cup sugar
1-tablespoon flour
1-teaspoon vanilla extract
½ cup nonfat sour cream
2 egg whites
½ cup graham-cracker crumbs
1 pint sliced strawberries

1.   Blend first four ingredients with electric mixer at
      medium speed. Blend in sour cream and egg whites.

2.   Spray 9-inch pie-pan with nonfat cooking spray;
      sprinkle with crumbs.

3.   Pour in cheese mixture, and bake at 325 degrees F for
      about 40 minutes.

4.   Cool, then refrigerate for around 3 hours. Top with
      berries and serve

      This is really tasty for such a light recipe. Try it and
I'm sure you will agree.

ACKNOWLEDGMENTS

This book owes its existence to a number of people…

My son and personal trainer, Ryan Haines, for guiding me to a healthier, happier life.

Judith A. Habert, Publisher/Editor-in-Chief of San Diego Woman magazine, who has encouraged and supported me throughout this process, and has taught me so much about writing.

The members of my writing group, Diane Netter, Judi Snyder, and Robin Pickett, whose feedback, and editing were invaluable.

My son/marketing consultant, Aaron Haines, who convinced me many people would want to read my book, and showed me how to reach them.

My cycle instructor, Stacy Becker, for her interest, suggestions, and encouragement.

Patti C. Dietz, great cook, wine maker and long time friend, for some of the delicious recipes I have included in this book.

My husband and number one fan, Mark Haines, for his undying belief in this project.